DEVELOPING LEADERSHIP SKILLS FOR EFFECTIVE RESPIRATORY CARE MANAGEMENT

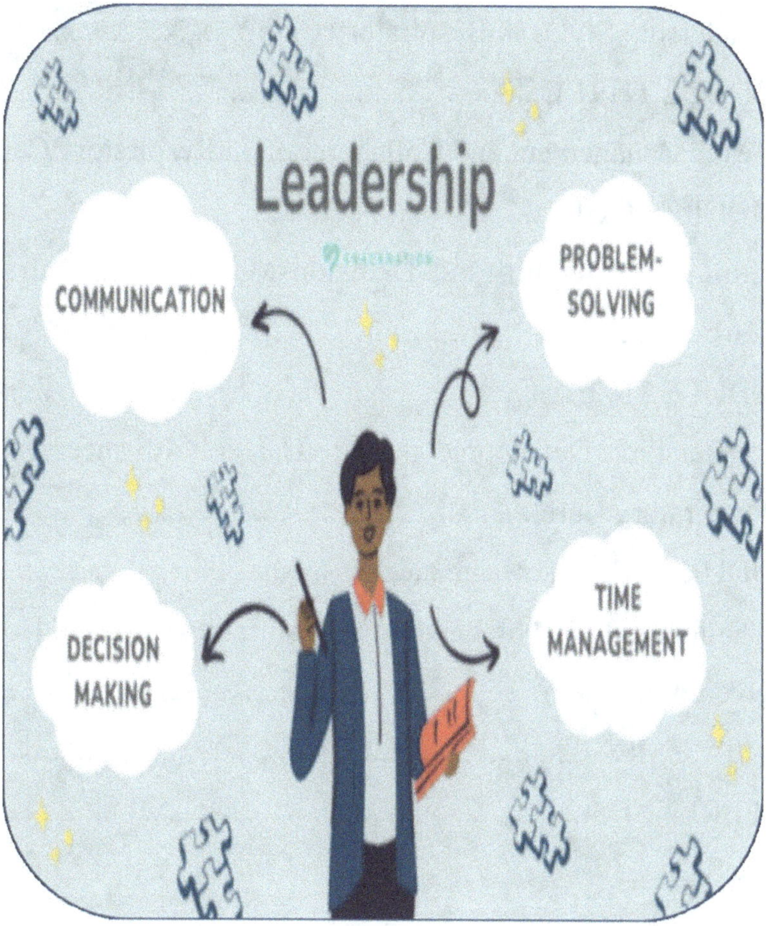

Table of Contents

COURSE OVERVIEW

This course is designed to equip respiratory care professionals with essential leadership and management skills. Participants will explore key principles of healthcare leadership, decision-making strategies, communication techniques, and best practices for managing respiratory care teams effectively. By the end of the course, healthcare providers will have the knowledge and confidence to lead their teams, improve patient outcomes, and contribute to the advancement of respiratory care services.

COURSE OBJECTIVE

The objective of this course is to equip respiratory care professionals with essential leadership skills to effectively manage teams, make informed decisions, and navigate challenges in healthcare settings. Participants will explore leadership theories, communication strategies, ethical decision-making, and team management techniques, enabling them to enhance patient care, foster collaboration, and advance their careers in respiratory therapy.

INTRODUCTION

Leadership in respiratory care is more than just managing a team it is about guiding, inspiring, and advocating for both patients and healthcare professionals. Respiratory therapists (RTs) play a crucial role in healthcare, providing life-saving interventions, supporting patients with chronic and acute respiratory conditions, and working alongside interdisciplinary teams in high-pressure environments. As the field of respiratory care evolves, effective leadership becomes increasingly essential for improving patient outcomes, enhancing team performance, and navigating the challenges of modern healthcare.

This book is designed to provide respiratory therapists whether new to leadership or seasoned professionals with the knowledge, skills, and strategies needed to become strong and effective leaders in their field. From understanding the core principles of leadership to exploring different leadership styles, managing teams, and making ethical decisions, this book offers a comprehensive guide to mastering the art of leadership in respiratory care.

In a profession where every second counts, strong leadership can mean the difference between success and failure in critical situations. Leadership in respiratory care is not just about holding a title; it is about taking initiative, making informed decisions, and fostering a collaborative environment where all team members feel empowered to provide the best possible care. Whether in hospitals, clinics, rehabilitation centers, or home healthcare settings, respiratory therapists who embrace leadership can drive positive change, improve workplace culture, and advocate for advancements in patient care.

Great leadership is not something you are born with it is a skill that can be learned, practiced, and refined over time. By equipping yourself with the knowledge and strategies in this book, you will be better prepared to lead your team, advocate for patients, and make a meaningful impact in the field of respiratory care.

Let's begin the journey toward becoming an effective and inspiring leader in respiratory care.

MODULE ONE

DEFINITION OF LEADERSHIP IN HEALTHCARE

Leadership in healthcare is the ability to influence, guide, and inspire individuals or teams toward achieving a common goal in patient care and organizational success. It involves decision-making, strategic planning, communication, and fostering a culture of teamwork and innovation. Unlike traditional leadership in other industries, healthcare leadership requires a deep understanding of clinical expertise, ethical considerations, and the ability to navigate complex medical and administrative environments.

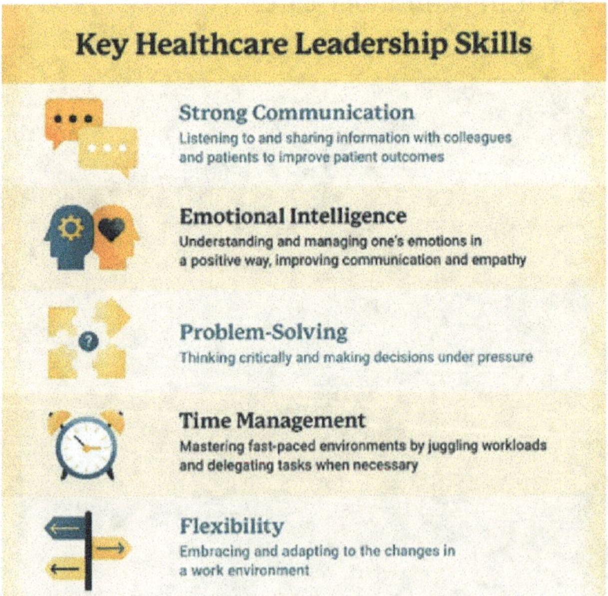
Key Healthcare Leadership Skills
Strong Communication
Listening to and sharing information with colleagues and patients to improve patient outcomes
Emotional Intelligence
Understanding and managing one's emotions in a positive way, improving communication and empathy
Problem-Solving
Thinking critically and making decisions under pressure
Time Management
Mastering fast-paced environments by juggling workloads and delegating tasks when necessary
Flexibility
Embracing and adapting to the changes in a work environment

In the context of respiratory care, leadership extends beyond supervising teams. It includes advocating for patient-centered care, promoting best practices in respiratory therapy, and guiding healthcare teams through challenging situations such as emergencies, policy changes, and technological advancements. Respiratory care leaders must possess both clinical expertise and the ability to motivate and influence their peers toward delivering optimal patient care.

IMPORTANCE OF LEADERSHIP IN RESPIRATORY CARE

Leadership in respiratory care is crucial for multiple reasons, including patient safety, efficient healthcare delivery, and the professional growth of respiratory therapists (RTs). Effective leadership ensures that RTs are well-equipped to handle critical situations, implement evidence-based practices, and contribute to interdisciplinary teams.

1. Enhancing Patient Outcomes: Leaders in respiratory care advocate for high-quality treatment plans, adherence to protocols, and continuous improvement in patient care. They help ensure patients receive the best respiratory support, whether in intensive care units (ICUs), emergency departments, or home-based settings.

2. Driving Innovation and Best Practices: Healthcare is constantly evolving, with new technologies, treatments, and research influencing respiratory therapy. Strong leadership fosters an environment where RTs can embrace innovations, such as non-invasive ventilation, advanced life support, and pulmonary rehabilitation techniques.
3. Improving Teamwork and Collaboration: Respiratory therapists often work alongside physicians, nurses, and other healthcare professionals. Leaders facilitate effective communication and collaboration among these groups, ensuring seamless patient care transitions and preventing medical errors.
4. Ensuring Compliance and Ethical Practice: Healthcare leaders ensure that respiratory care practices align with regulatory standards, institutional policies, and ethical guidelines. They advocate for patient rights, infection control measures, and the responsible use of medical resources.
5. Supporting Professional Growth and Development: Strong leaders mentor and support respiratory therapists, encouraging professional development through continuing education, certifications, and specialized

training. This not only benefits individual therapists but also strengthens the entire respiratory care field.

KEY TRAITS OF EFFECTIVE HEALTHCARE LEADERS

Effective leadership in respiratory care requires a combination of technical knowledge, interpersonal skills, and emotional intelligence. Some of the essential traits include:

1. Communication Skills: Clear and effective communication is vital in healthcare. Leaders must convey complex medical information to patients, collaborate with multidisciplinary teams, and provide constructive feedback to their staff.
2. Emotional Intelligence: Understanding and managing emotions, both one's own and others', is crucial for building strong relationships and fostering a supportive work environment. Leaders with high emotional intelligence can resolve conflicts, motivate their teams, and handle stressful situations with composure.
3. Critical Thinking and Decision-Making: Respiratory care often involves making quick, life-saving decisions. Leaders must analyze situations, weigh risks, and make informed choices that prioritize patient safety and quality of care.

4. Adaptability and Resilience: The healthcare landscape is constantly changing. Leaders must be flexible and open to new protocols, technological advancements, and unexpected challenges, such as pandemics or hospital crises.
5. Integrity and Ethical Leadership: Ethical decision-making is fundamental in healthcare. Leaders must adhere to the highest ethical standards, advocate for patient rights, and set an example of professionalism and accountability.
6. Inspirational and Motivational Abilities: An effective leader inspires their team by setting a positive example, recognizing achievements, and fostering a culture of learning and improvement.

DIFFERENCE BETWEEN LEADERSHIP AND MANAGEMENT

While leadership and management are often used interchangeably, they have distinct roles in healthcare:

Aspect	Leadership	Management
Focus	Vision, inspiration, and innovation	Execution, organization, and control
Approach	People-oriented, motivating teams	Task-oriented, ensuring efficiency
Decision making	Long-term strategic thinking	Short-term operational execution
Change	Drives and embraces change	Maintains stability and order
Role in respiratory care	Advocates for patient-centered care and new protocols	Ensures daily operations and adherence to policies

Both leadership and management are necessary in respiratory care. Managers ensure the smooth operation of departments, while leaders inspire and guide teams toward continuous improvement and excellence in patient care.

THE ROLE OF RESPIRATORY THERAPISTS AS LEADERS

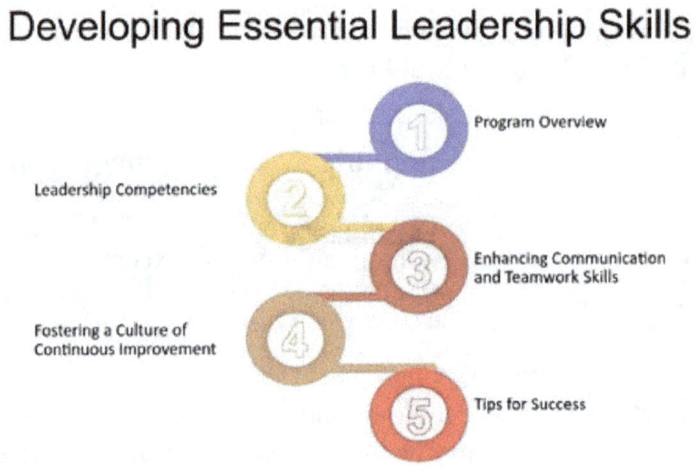

Respiratory therapists (RTs) play a crucial role in patient care, and many find themselves in leadership positions, even if they are not formally designated as leaders. Their expertise, ability to work under pressure, and interactions with patients and other healthcare professionals place them in positions of influence. Here are key ways RTs serve as leaders:

1. Advocating for Patients: RTs ensure that patients receive the best respiratory care, educate them about their conditions, and advocate for necessary interventions, such as mechanical ventilation, oxygen therapy, or pulmonary rehabilitation.
2. Guiding and Mentoring New Therapists: Experienced RTs often train and mentor new hires, helping them

develop clinical skills and confidence in high-stakes environments like the ICU or emergency department.

3. Implementing Evidence-Based Practices: Leaders in respiratory care stay updated on the latest research and integrate new techniques and technologies into their practice to improve patient outcomes.
4. Participating in Policy Development: RTs contribute to hospital and national respiratory care policies, ensuring protocols align with best practices and patient needs.
5. Crisis Management and Decision-Making: During emergencies, such as cardiac arrests, respiratory failures, or pandemics, RTs must act decisively and lead resuscitation or ventilation strategies.
6. Promoting a Collaborative Healthcare Environment: RTs work closely with physicians, nurses, and other healthcare professionals to ensure cohesive patient care, bridging communication gaps and facilitating effective teamwork.
7. Engaging in Continuing Education and Professional Development: Great leaders never stop learning. RTs who pursue further certifications, attend conferences, and stay informed about advancements in respiratory therapy position themselves as leaders in their field.

Leadership in respiratory care is not just about holding a title, it's about making a difference in patient outcomes, improving healthcare efficiency, and guiding fellow professionals toward excellence. Whether through advocacy, mentorship, policy development, or clinical expertise, respiratory therapists have numerous opportunities to lead and influence their field. Developing strong leadership skills ensures that RTs remain at the forefront of patient care and innovation in respiratory therapy.

DISCUSSION QUESTIONS:

What are the key leadership traits that respiratory therapists should develop?

How does leadership differ from management in a healthcare setting?

MODULE TWO

LEADERSHIP STYLES IN RESPIRATORY CARE

Leadership in respiratory care is a dynamic and evolving concept. Effective leadership goes beyond just managing a team; it involves inspiring, guiding, and adapting to the needs of both patients and healthcare professionals. Different leadership styles can significantly impact the quality of care, team performance, and overall workplace culture. Understanding these styles and knowing when to apply them can make a significant difference in patient outcomes and team dynamics.

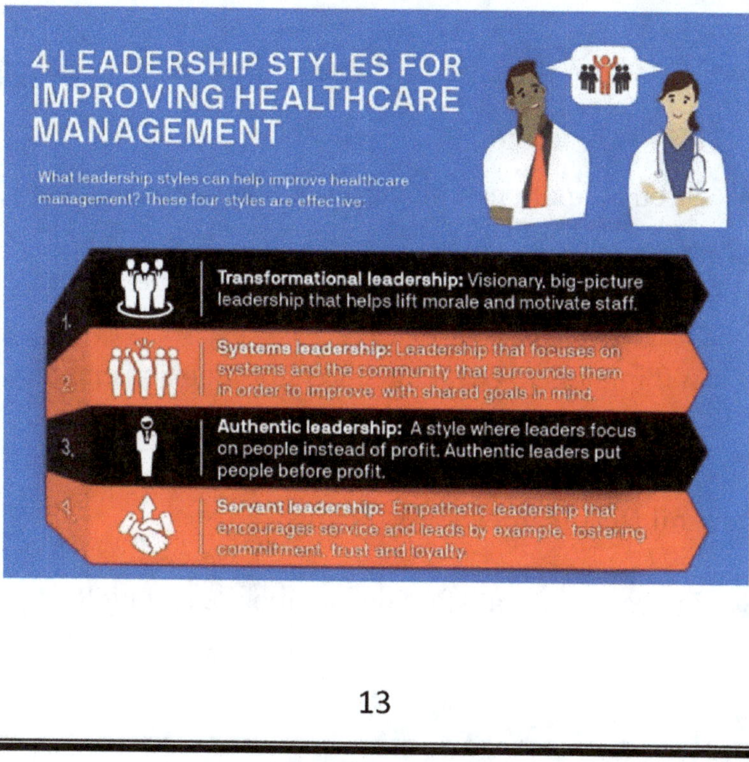

This module will explore various leadership styles commonly found in healthcare, their effects on respiratory care teams, and how respiratory therapists (RTs) can identify and adapt their leadership styles to different situations.

OVERVIEW OF DIFFERENT LEADERSHIP STYLES

1. Transformational Leadership

Transformational leadership is one of the most effective styles in healthcare. It focuses on inspiring and motivating team members to achieve their highest potential. Leaders using this style foster innovation, encourage professional development, and create a vision that guides the entire team.

Characteristics of Transformational Leaders

- Visionary thinking and the ability to see the bigger picture
- Strong emotional intelligence, including empathy and communication skills
- Encouragement of teamwork and collaboration
- Willingness to challenge the status quo and embrace new ideas

Impact on Respiratory Care Teams

- Increased job satisfaction and morale among RTs

- Higher levels of patient-centered care due to motivated employees
- Encourages a learning culture where RTs can grow professionally

Example in Respiratory Care

An RT supervisor who implements weekly training sessions to keep the team updated on new treatments and technologies is demonstrating transformational leadership. By motivating the team and setting high expectations, they create a positive work environment that benefits both staff and patients.

2. **Transactional Leadership**

Transactional leadership is based on a structured system of rewards and punishments. This style focuses on efficiency, compliance, and maintaining order within the organization.

Characteristics of Transactional Leaders

- Focus on clear roles and responsibilities
- Use of performance-based rewards and consequences
- Emphasis on following protocols and regulations

Impact on Respiratory Care Teams

- Ensures that RTs follow established procedures and guidelines

- Provides clear expectations and accountability
- May limit creativity and innovation if overused

Example in Respiratory Care

A respiratory department manager who rewards staff for achieving high patient satisfaction scores while enforcing strict adherence to infection control protocols is using a transactional leadership approach. This can be effective in maintaining high standards of care but may need to be balanced with other leadership styles to avoid rigidity.

3. **Democratic Leadership**

Democratic leadership, also known as participative leadership, involves including team members in decision-making. It fosters a sense of ownership, encourages collaboration, and values input from all team members.

Characteristics of Democratic Leaders

- Open communication and active listening
- Encouragement of teamwork and shared decision-making
- Valuing diverse perspectives and ideas

Impact on Respiratory Care Teams

- Boosts morale and job satisfaction by giving RTs a voice

- Encourages innovation and problem-solving within the team
- Can slow decision-making in high-pressure situations

Example in Respiratory Care

An RT director who regularly holds team meetings to discuss new protocols and allows staff to provide feedback before implementation demonstrates democratic leadership. This ensures that frontline workers have input, leading to better adherence to changes.

4. Autocratic Leadership

Autocratic leadership is a top-down approach where decisions are made by the leader without consulting the team. This style is most effective in emergency or high-risk situations where quick decision-making is essential.

Characteristics of Autocratic Leaders

- High level of control and authority
- Clear, direct instructions with little room for discussion
- Focus on efficiency and quick decision-making

Impact on Respiratory Care Teams

- Useful in crisis situations where immediate action is required

- Can create a highly structured environment, reducing uncertainty
- May lead to low morale if overused, as employees feel unheard

Example in Respiratory Care

In a hospital's ICU, a lead RT giving direct orders during a patient's respiratory failure event is using an autocratic leadership style. In this scenario, clear direction and immediate action are critical to saving lives. However, if used outside of emergencies, this style can discourage teamwork.

5. Servant Leadership

Servant leadership focuses on serving the needs of the team rather than exercising authority. Leaders prioritize team members' well-being and professional development while fostering a supportive and compassionate work environment.

Characteristics of Servant Leaders

- Commitment to the growth and well-being of their team
- Strong emphasis on empathy and listening
- Prioritization of team needs over personal authority

Impact on Respiratory Care Teams

- Creates a strong sense of community and trust

- Encourages professional growth and mentorship
- Can be time-consuming and may not work well in highly structured environments

Example in Respiratory Care

A senior RT who mentors new staff, ensures work-life balance for their team, and advocates for better working conditions embodies servant leadership. By putting the team's well-being first, they create a supportive and productive work environment.

HOW DIFFERENT LEADERSHIP STYLES IMPACT HEALTHCARE TEAMS

Each leadership style affects respiratory care teams differently. While transformational and servant leadership styles often create a positive work culture, transactional and autocratic leadership are essential for maintaining structure and compliance. Democratic leadership fosters innovation but may slow decision-making, and servant leadership builds trust but requires time and commitment.

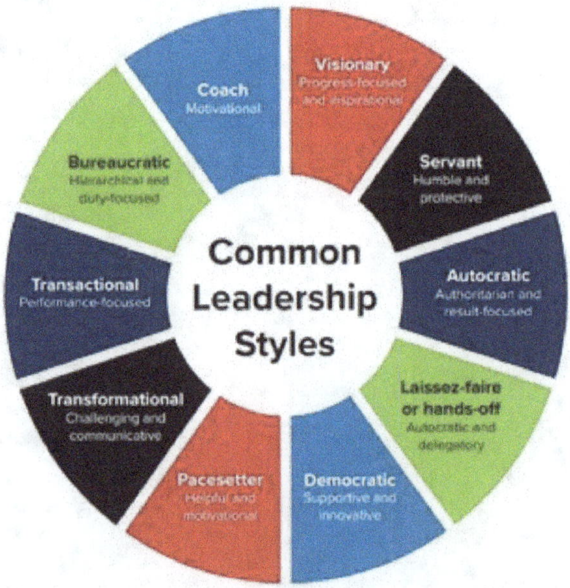
Common Leadership Styles
Visionary
Progress-focused and inspirational
Servant
Humble and protective
Autocratic
Authoritarian and result-focused
Laissez-faire or hands-off
Autocratic and delegatory
Democratic
Supportive and innovative
Pacesetter
Helpful and motivational
Transformational
Challenging and communicative
Transactional
Performance-focused
Bureaucratic
Hierarchical and duty-focused
Coach
Motivational

Indeed https://www.indeed.com/career-advice/career-development/10-common-leadership-styles

An effective respiratory care leader understands when to use different styles based on the team's needs and the situation at hand.

IDENTIFYING YOUR LEADERSHIP STYLE

Understanding your leadership style is crucial for personal and professional growth. Here are some steps to help you determine your leadership style:

- Self-Assessment – Reflect on how you naturally lead others. Do you prefer collaboration, structure, or inspiring change?
- Feedback from Colleagues – Ask peers and supervisors how they perceive your leadership approach.
- Situational Analysis – Consider past experiences where you had to take charge. What methods did you use?
- Personality and Strengths Tests – Tools like the Myers-Briggs Type Indicator (MBTI) or the Leadership Style Questionnaire can help identify tendencies.

WHEN TO ADAPT DIFFERENT LEADERSHIP STYLES IN RESPIRATORY CARE

Flexibility in leadership is key to success in healthcare. Different situations require different leadership approaches. Here's when to apply each style:

- Transformational Leadership – When introducing new policies, technologies, or initiatives that require team buy-in and motivation.

- Transactional Leadership – When strict adherence to protocols is necessary, such as infection control or compliance with hospital regulations.
- Democratic Leadership – When making long-term changes, such as adjusting workflow procedures, to ensure all team members have input.
- Autocratic Leadership – During high-pressure situations, such as patient emergencies, where immediate decisions are required.
- Servant Leadership – When mentoring new RTs or advocating for better working conditions within the department.

By mastering the ability to shift between leadership styles based on the situation, respiratory care leaders can create a more effective, engaged, and resilient healthcare team.

Leadership in respiratory care is not one-size-fits-all. Each leadership style has its benefits and drawbacks, and successful leaders know when to apply the appropriate style. By understanding these different approaches, respiratory therapists can become more effective leaders, improving both patient outcomes and workplace dynamics.

Identifying and adapting leadership styles is a continuous learning process, but with self-awareness, experience, and education, RTs can strengthen their leadership skills and make a lasting impact in their field.

DISCUSSION QUESTIONS:

Which leadership style do you think works best in respiratory care, and why?

How can a respiratory therapist adapt their leadership style to different team members?

MODULE THREE

TEAM MANAGEMENT AND COLLABORATION IN RESPIRATORY CARE

Effective team management and collaboration are essential in respiratory care, where patient outcomes often depend on seamless teamwork. Respiratory therapists (RTs) work in fast-paced, high-stakes environments alongside physicians, nurses, and other healthcare professionals. Strong leadership ensures that teams function efficiently, communicate effectively, and remain motivated to provide the best care possible.

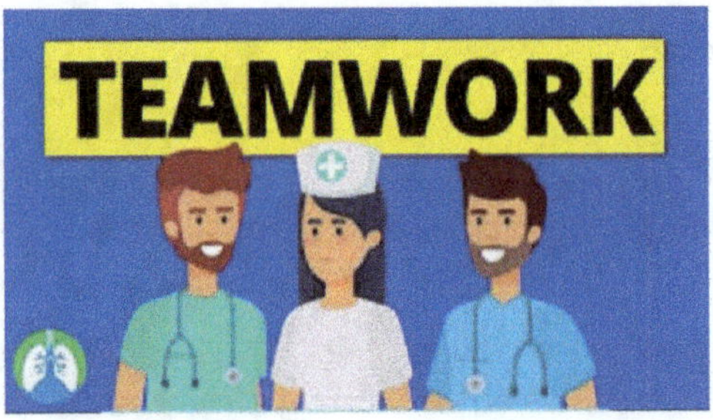

This module will explore the fundamentals of building and leading a successful respiratory care team, encouraging interprofessional collaboration, empowering team members, delegating responsibilities, and handling challenges that arise in a healthcare setting.

BUILDING AND LEADING AN EFFECTIVE RESPIRATORY CARE TEAM

A well-structured team is the backbone of high-quality patient care. A successful respiratory care team consists of professionals with diverse skills who work toward a shared goal: improving patient health. Leaders in respiratory care must build teams that are skilled, cohesive, and adaptable.

Key Steps to Building an Effective Team:

1. Define Roles and Responsibilities

Every team member should have a clear understanding of their role. RTs may specialize in critical care, neonatal care, pulmonary rehabilitation, or sleep medicine. Ensuring that everyone knows their specific duties reduces confusion and enhances efficiency.

2. Hire and Retain Talented Professionals

Recruiting RTs with the right qualifications and mindset is crucial. Beyond technical skills, successful RTs must have strong communication abilities, empathy, and teamwork skills. Retaining top talent requires fostering a positive work environment and offering professional development opportunities.

3. Establish a Positive Work Culture

A team thrives in an environment where respect, open communication, and collaboration are encouraged. Leaders should set the tone by promoting inclusivity and valuing diverse perspectives.

4. Set Clear Goals and Expectations

Establishing clear performance standards and expectations keeps the team aligned with organizational objectives. Leaders should regularly communicate goals and provide feedback to ensure continuous improvement.

5. Encourage Continuous Learning

Providing ongoing training and mentorship opportunities allows RTs to expand their skills and stay updated on new technologies and treatment methods. This fosters professional growth and enhances team competence.

ENCOURAGING TEAMWORK AND INTERPROFESSIONAL COLLABORATION

Healthcare is a multidisciplinary field, and respiratory therapists frequently work with nurses, physicians, physical therapists, and other professionals. Effective collaboration is crucial to delivering comprehensive patient care.

Strategies to Foster Collaboration:

1. Promote Open Communication

Clear and open communication ensures that all team members are on the same page. Encouraging team members to voice concerns, ask questions, and share insights can prevent misunderstandings and errors. Tools like electronic health records (EHRs) and shared communication platforms (e.g., Slack, Microsoft Teams) can improve information exchange.

2. Encourage Mutual Respect and Trust

Teams function best when members respect each other's expertise. Leaders should emphasize that every role in the healthcare system is vital and encourage a culture of mutual support.

3. Hold Regular Team Meetings and Case Discussions

Routine meetings allow RTs to collaborate with other professionals, review patient cases, and develop treatment strategies. These discussions can enhance patient care by leveraging collective knowledge and expertise.

4. Use Interdisciplinary Training and Simulations

Conducting training sessions and medical simulations that involve multiple healthcare disciplines helps professionals understand each other's roles and responsibilities. This strengthens teamwork and improves coordination during real-life medical situations.

5. Address and Resolve Conflicts Early

Disagreements are inevitable in high-pressure environments. Leaders must mediate conflicts swiftly, ensuring that differences do not disrupt team harmony or patient care. Conflict resolution training can help team members navigate disputes constructively.

MOTIVATING AND EMPOWERING TEAM MEMBERS

A motivated team delivers better patient care, exhibits higher job satisfaction, and experiences lower burnout rates. Leaders in respiratory care must find ways to inspire and empower their teams.

Ways to Motivate and Empower RTs:

1. Recognize and Reward Contributions

Acknowledging hard work boosts morale and encourages continued excellence. Public recognition, employee of the month programs, and performance-based incentives can help motivate team members.

2. Provide Opportunities for Growth

Offering continuing education, mentorship, and leadership training allows RTs to advance their careers. Leaders should support team members who seek professional certifications, attend conferences, or pursue advanced degrees.

3. Encourage Autonomy and Decision-Making

Allowing RTs to make decisions within their scope of practice fosters confidence and engagement. Empowered professionals take greater ownership of their roles and contribute more effectively to patient care.

4. Support Work-Life Balance

Overworked teams experience higher levels of stress and burnout. Implementing fair scheduling, encouraging breaks, and offering mental health resources help maintain a healthy work environment.

5. Create a Sense of Purpose

Reminding RTs of their vital role in saving lives and improving patient health reinforces their sense of purpose. Leaders should highlight success stories and the positive impact of their work.

DELEGATION AND WORKLOAD DISTRIBUTION

Delegation is a crucial leadership skill in respiratory care. Leaders must distribute workloads efficiently to prevent burnout and ensure that tasks are completed effectively.

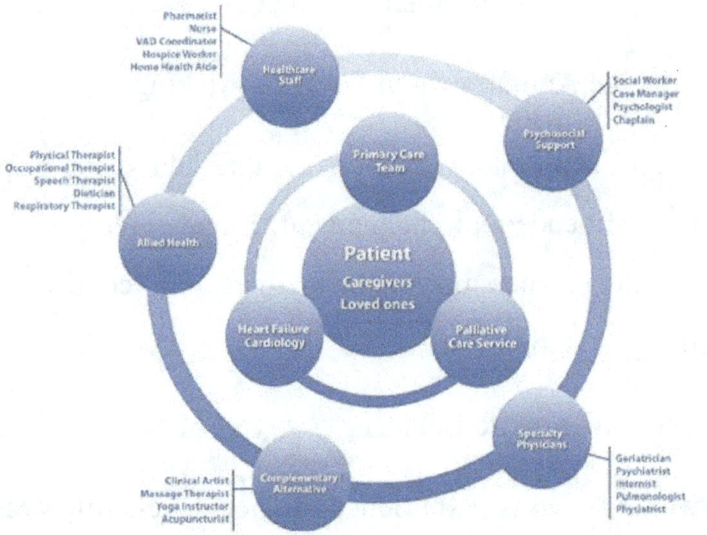

Principles of Effective Delegation:

1. Match Tasks to Team Member Strengths

Assign tasks based on team members' expertise and experience. Senior RTs may handle complex cases, while newer RTs can take on routine procedures under supervision.

2. Clearly Define Expectations

Delegation should come with clear instructions, objectives, and deadlines. Unclear expectations can lead to errors and inefficiencies.

3. Encourage Teamwork in Delegation

Delegation should not feel like an uneven burden. Encouraging a team-based approach where members support each other fosters a collaborative work environment.

4. Monitor and Provide Feedback

Checking in on delegated tasks ensures quality control. Leaders should provide constructive feedback and guidance to improve future performance.

5. Empower and Trust Team Members

Micromanaging can hinder confidence and slow down workflow. Leaders should trust their team members to complete assigned tasks while remaining available for support if needed.

HANDLING TEAM CHALLENGES

Every team faces challenges, and leaders must be equipped to navigate them effectively. Some common challenges in respiratory care teams include:

1. High-Stress Work Environment

Respiratory care professionals often work in high-pressure settings, especially in ICUs and emergency departments.

Solution: Promote stress management strategies, ensure adequate staffing, and provide mental health resources.

2. Staff Shortages and Burnout

A shortage of RTs can lead to increased workloads, exhaustion, and decreased job satisfaction.

Solution: Advocate for better staffing ratios, offer overtime incentives, and implement wellness programs.

3. Resistance to Change

Some team members may resist new protocols, technology, or leadership approaches.

Solution: Involve staff in decision-making, provide adequate training, and explain the benefits of changes to gain buy-in.

4. Communication Barriers

Miscommunication can lead to errors, misunderstandings, and tension within the team.

Solution: Encourage active listening, use structured handoff reports, and implement clear communication protocols.

5. Conflict Among Team Members

Disagreements can disrupt team harmony and affect patient care.

Solution: Address conflicts quickly and fairly, promote open dialogue, and use conflict resolution techniques to maintain a positive work environment.

Effective team management and collaboration are essential for providing high-quality respiratory care. Building a strong team, fostering interprofessional collaboration, motivating and empowering staff, delegating tasks wisely, and managing challenges all contribute to a positive and productive work environment. Leaders who prioritize these elements ensure better patient outcomes, improved job satisfaction, and a resilient respiratory care team.

DISCUSSION QUESTIONS:

What are some challenges in managing a respiratory care team, and how can leaders address them?

How can respiratory care leaders foster a collaborative work environment?

MODULE FOUR

ETHICAL LEADERSHIP AND DECISION-MAKING IN RESPIRATORY CARE

Ethical leadership in respiratory care is critical to ensuring that patient-centered care aligns with professional integrity, legal standards, and moral responsibility. Respiratory therapists (RTs) often face challenging situations requiring difficult decisions, such as end-of-life care, informed consent, patient autonomy, and resource allocation. Ethical leadership helps guide these decisions by balancing medical necessity, patient rights, and institutional policies.

Components of Ethical Decision-Making

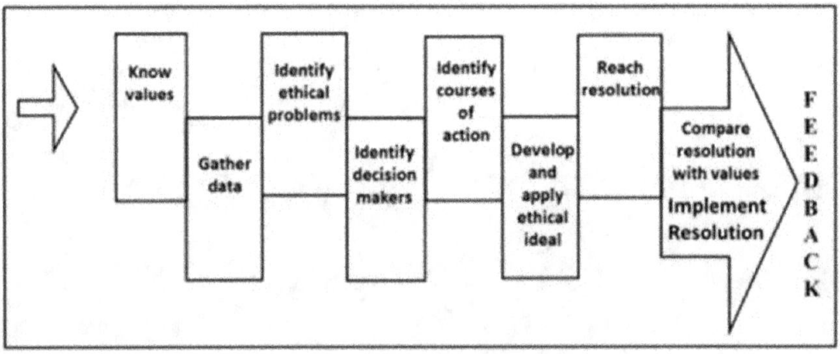

This module will explore ethical dilemmas in respiratory care, the role of ethics in decision-making, the application of ethical principles in leadership, and real-world case studies demonstrating ethical leadership in action.

UNDERSTANDING ETHICAL DILEMMAS IN RESPIRATORY CARE

An ethical dilemma arises when a healthcare professional must choose between two or more morally acceptable or conflicting options. In respiratory care, these dilemmas can be particularly complex because respiratory therapists work in critical care settings, where life-or-death decisions often need to be made quickly.

Common Ethical Dilemmas in Respiratory Care

1. End-of-Life Decisions and Withholding Treatment

RTs frequently work with patients on ventilators and other life-sustaining devices. When a patient is terminally ill or has no chance of recovery, the question arises: Should mechanical ventilation be continued, or should life support be withdrawn?

The dilemma intensifies if the patient has no advance directive and family members disagree on treatment decisions.

2. Patient Autonomy vs. Medical Best Interest

Patients have the right to refuse treatment, even if doing so may result in death or severe complications. For example, a patient with severe chronic obstructive pulmonary disease (COPD) might refuse intubation despite respiratory failure.

Ethical leaders must respect patient autonomy while also ensuring that patients fully understand the consequences of their decisions.

3. Informed Consent and Capacity to Decide

Some patients, such as those with dementia or impaired cognitive function, may not have the capacity to make informed decisions.

In cases where surrogate decision-makers are involved, conflicts may arise if the surrogate's choices contradict what the medical team believes is in the patient's best interest.

4. Allocation of Limited Resources

In times of crisis, such as during a pandemic or natural disaster, hospitals may experience shortages of ventilators, oxygen, or staff.

Ethical leaders must make difficult decisions about who receives life-saving treatments when resources are scarce.

5. Conflicts of Interest and Professional Integrity

RTs may face pressure from hospital administration to discharge patients quickly to free up beds, even when it may not be in the best interest of the patient.

Ethical leadership requires balancing institutional priorities with the duty to provide quality care.

THE ROLE OF ETHICS IN DECISION-MAKING

Ethical decision-making in respiratory care requires a structured approach that prioritizes patient well-being while considering legal and professional standards. Leaders must cultivate an ethical culture within their teams by fostering open discussions about moral dilemmas and ensuring that ethical considerations are part of the decision-making process.

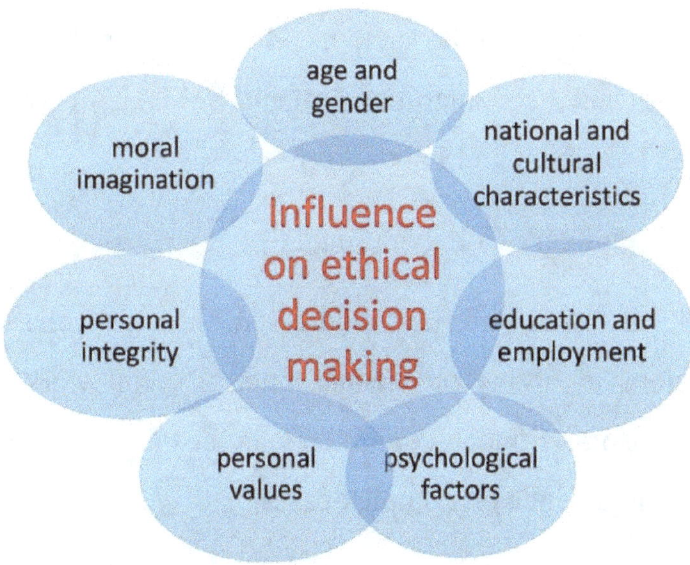
Influence on ethical decision making
age and gender
national and cultural characteristics
education and employment
psychological factors
personal values
personal integrity
moral imagination

Key Factors Influencing Ethical Decision-Making

1. Medical Ethics Principles

Ethical decisions in healthcare are guided by four fundamental principles:

- Autonomy – Respecting patients' rights to make their own healthcare decisions.
- Beneficence – Acting in the best interest of the patient to promote well-being.
- Non-Maleficence – Avoiding harm to the patient.
- Justice – Ensuring fair and equitable treatment for all patients.

2. Institutional Policies and Legal Guidelines

Ethical decisions must comply with hospital policies, state laws, and federal regulations such as HIPAA (Health Insurance Portability and Accountability Act) and EMTALA (Emergency Medical Treatment and Labor Act).

3. Interdisciplinary Collaboration

Ethical dilemmas are best addressed through collaborative discussions involving physicians, nurses, social workers, and legal advisors. Ethical committees in hospitals can provide additional guidance on complex cases.

4. Cultural and Religious Considerations

Patients come from diverse backgrounds with different beliefs about medical interventions, end-of-life care, and organ donation. Ethical leaders must navigate these differences sensitively while ensuring that care remains patient-centered.

5. Communication and Transparency

Open, honest communication with patients and families is essential in ethical decision-making. Explaining treatment options, potential risks, and ethical concerns helps build trust and prevent misunderstandings.

APPLYING ETHICAL PRINCIPLES IN LEADERSHIP

Ethical leadership in respiratory care means leading by example, fostering a culture of integrity, and ensuring that ethical considerations guide daily practices.

Characteristics of an Ethical Leader in Respiratory Care

1. Integrity and Honesty

Ethical leaders do not compromise on patient care, even when facing external pressures. They uphold professional and moral standards at all times.

2. Empathy and Compassion

Understanding patients' and families' emotional struggles helps leaders make humane decisions. Ethical leaders listen to concerns, validate emotions, and provide compassionate care.

3. Advocacy for Patients' Rights

Ethical leaders advocate for patients, ensuring that their voices are heard in medical decisions. They help patients and families understand their rights and options.

4. Commitment to Fairness and Justice

Leaders must ensure that every patient receives equal treatment, regardless of socioeconomic status, race, or personal background.

5. Encouraging Ethical Awareness in Teams

Ethical leadership involves creating a workplace culture where team members feel comfortable discussing ethical dilemmas. Leaders should facilitate training sessions, encourage ethical case discussions, and provide resources on medical ethics.

CASE STUDIES ON ETHICAL LEADERSHIP IN RESPIRATORY CARE

Case Study 1: The Dilemma of Withdrawing Life Support

Scenario:

A 72-year-old patient with advanced-stage lung cancer is on a ventilator. The family is divided—some want to continue life support, while others wish to follow the patient's previous verbal wishes to withdraw treatment.

Ethical Issues:

- Patient autonomy vs. family decision-making
- Determining the patient's best interest
- Emotional distress of healthcare providers

Ethical Leadership Approach:

The respiratory care team consults the hospital ethics committee.

- A family meeting is held to discuss the patient's prognosis, potential suffering, and possible outcomes.
- The leader ensures that decisions align with the patient's best interest while respecting family perspectives.

Case Study 2: A COVID-19 Ventilator Shortage

Scenario:

During a COVID-19 surge, a hospital has a limited number of ventilators, but several critically ill patients need them. A young patient with a high survival chance and an elderly patient with multiple comorbidities both require ventilation.

Ethical Issues:

- Resource allocation and triage decisions
- Justice and fairness in patient care
- Emotional burden on healthcare staff

Ethical Leadership Approach:

- The team follows established triage protocols to determine ventilator allocation based on medical evidence rather than subjective bias.
- The leader ensures transparency in decision-making and provides emotional support to staff struggling with the moral burden.

Case Study 3: A Patient's Refusal of Treatment

Scenario:

A middle-aged COPD patient arrives at the hospital in respiratory distress but refuses intubation due to personal beliefs. The medical team believes intubation could save his life, but the patient insists on comfort care.

Ethical Issues:

- Patient autonomy vs. medical judgment
- Ensuring informed consent
- The role of family in decision-making

Ethical Leadership Approach:

- The leader facilitates an in-depth discussion with the patient, ensuring he understands the consequences of refusing treatment.
- The patient's autonomy is respected, and comfort care is provided per his wishes.
- The team receives emotional support and debriefing after the case.

Ethical leadership in respiratory care requires a commitment to patient-centered values, moral integrity, and transparent decision-making. Leaders must navigate complex ethical dilemmas by applying ethical principles, encouraging open discussions, and ensuring fairness and compassion in all decisions. By fostering a strong ethical culture, respiratory care leaders contribute to improved patient outcomes, team morale, and the overall quality of healthcare.

DISCUSSION QUESTIONS:

How can a leader balance ethical considerations with hospital policies?

What are some ethical challenges that respiratory care leaders might face?

MODULE FIVE

LEADERSHIP DEVELOPMENT AND CAREER ADVANCEMENT IN RESPIRATORY CARE

Leadership in respiratory care is not confined to managerial roles it is a mindset and a continuous process of growth, learning, and adaptation. Developing leadership skills enables respiratory therapists (RTs) to take on more responsibilities, contribute to positive patient outcomes, and shape the future of respiratory care.

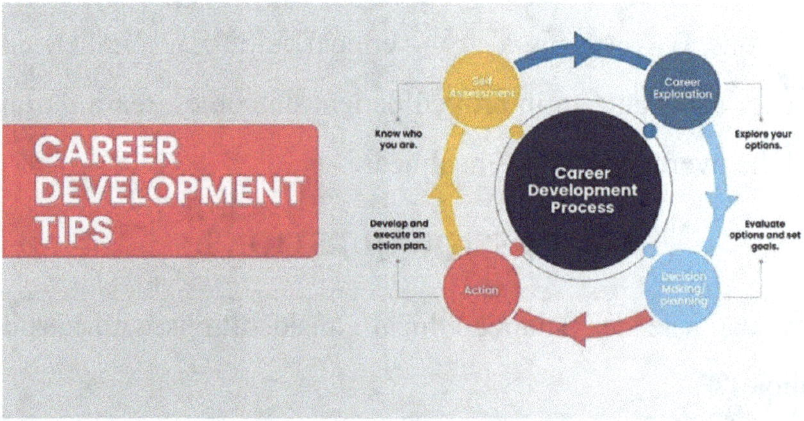

This module explores how RTs can develop leadership skills over time, the role of mentorship and professional development, career paths in respiratory care leadership, and strategies for setting personal and professional growth goals.

HOW TO DEVELOP LEADERSHIP SKILLS OVER TIME

Leadership is a skill that evolves with experience, self-awareness, and a commitment to continuous learning. Respiratory therapists can enhance their leadership abilities by engaging in structured education, seeking feedback, and taking on progressively greater responsibilities.

Key Strategies for Leadership Development

1. Gain Hands-On Experience

- Volunteering for leadership roles, such as team lead positions or participation in hospital committees, helps build confidence and decision-making skills.
- Supervising new RTs, students, or interns provides experience in mentorship and leadership.

2. Enhance Communication Skills

- Strong leaders communicate effectively with patients, families, and healthcare teams.
- Active listening, clear explanations, and the ability to handle difficult conversations are crucial skills to develop.

3. Pursue Continuing Education

- Attending leadership workshops, healthcare management courses, or obtaining advanced certifications (e.g.,

Certified Respiratory Therapist [CRT], Registered Respiratory Therapist [RRT], or specialized credentials like ACCS for adult critical care) enhances expertise.

- Earning a degree in healthcare administration, public health, or business administration provides a foundation for leadership roles.

4. Develop Critical Thinking and Problem-Solving Skills
   - Leaders must analyze complex situations, make informed decisions, and anticipate challenges before they arise.
   - Engaging in case studies, simulations, and leadership training exercises helps refine these skills.
5. Seek Constructive Feedback
   - Constructive feedback from supervisors, colleagues, and mentors allows RTs to identify areas for improvement.
   - Self-reflection through journaling or performance assessments also helps in personal growth.
6. Cultivate Emotional Intelligence
   - Leaders must manage their emotions and understand the emotions of others.
   - Emotional intelligence (EQ) includes self-awareness, empathy, adaptability, and conflict resolution skills.

7. Stay Informed on Industry Trends
    - Keeping up with advancements in respiratory therapy, healthcare policies, and technology ensures that leaders make informed decisions.
    - Reading medical journals, attending conferences, and participating in professional organizations (e.g., American Association for Respiratory Care [AARC]) help RTs stay current.

THE IMPORTANCE OF MENTORSHIP AND PROFESSIONAL DEVELOPMENT

Mentorship and professional development play a crucial role in shaping strong healthcare leaders. Respiratory therapists who engage in mentorship—whether as mentors or mentees—benefit from knowledge-sharing, networking, and career growth opportunities.

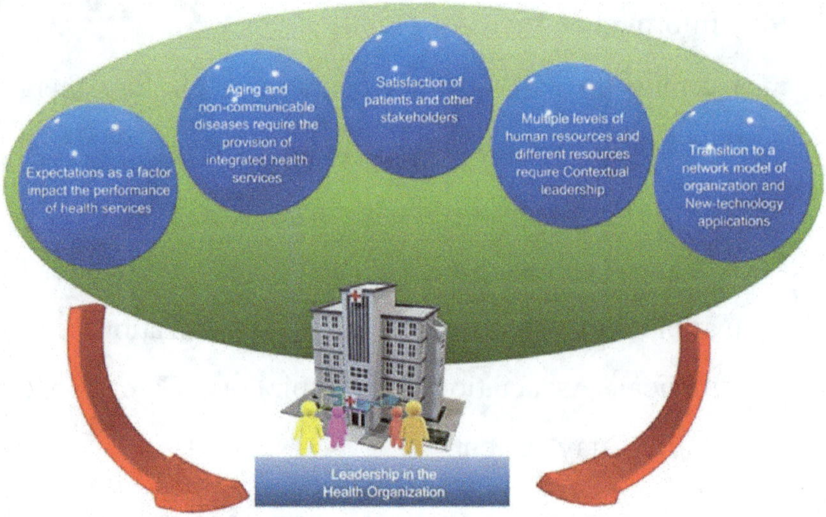

Benefits of Mentorship in Respiratory Care Leadership

1. Guidance and Career Support

Experienced mentors provide valuable insights into career advancement, workplace challenges, and leadership strategies.

Mentees gain access to new perspectives and industry connections.

2. Skill Development and Confidence Building

Mentors help RTs develop clinical expertise, decision-making skills, and professional confidence.

Having a trusted advisor fosters a sense of security when facing complex leadership challenges.

3. Networking Opportunities

Mentorship programs open doors to networking within hospital systems, professional organizations, and academic institutions.

Connections with healthcare leaders can lead to career advancements, job opportunities, and collaborations.

4. Fostering a Culture of Continuous Learning

Mentorship promotes lifelong learning and encourages both mentors and mentees to stay engaged in professional growth.

Hospitals and healthcare organizations with strong mentorship programs experience higher job satisfaction and retention rates.

HOW TO FIND A MENTOR IN RESPIRATORY CARE

- Professional Organizations: Joining groups like AARC or state respiratory therapy associations can help RTs connect with industry leaders.
- Workplace Programs: Many hospitals and clinics offer mentorship programs for career development.
- Educational Institutions: Professors, clinical instructors, and program directors can serve as mentors.
- Online Networking: Platforms like LinkedIn provide opportunities to connect with experienced respiratory care professionals.

CAREER PATHS IN RESPIRATORY CARE LEADERSHIP

Respiratory therapists have diverse career paths in leadership, ranging from clinical supervision to executive roles in healthcare administration. Understanding these career trajectories helps RTs set clear professional goals.

Common Leadership Roles in Respiratory Care

1. Lead Respiratory Therapist / Supervisor
   - Oversees daily operations in the respiratory care department.
   - Ensures staff adherence to protocols and policies.
   - Assists in training and onboarding new employees.
2. Respiratory Therapy Manager / Director
   - Manages staff schedules, budgets, and department policies.
   - Collaborates with hospital administrators to improve patient care.
   - Implements new respiratory care technologies and procedures.
3. Clinical Educator / Respiratory Therapy Instructor
   - Trains respiratory therapy students and new hires.
   - Develops educational programs and training materials.

- Conducts research and stays updated on the latest advancements in respiratory care.

4. Healthcare Administrator
   - Oversees hospital departments, including respiratory therapy services.
   - Focuses on financial management, policy-making, and operational efficiency.
   - Often requires additional education, such as a Master of Healthcare Administration (MHA).
5. Researcher or Clinical Specialist
   - Works in research institutions, medical device companies, or universities.
   - Develops new respiratory therapies, devices, and protocols.
   - Contributes to scientific advancements in respiratory care.
6. Entrepreneur / Consultant
   - Starts a respiratory therapy-related business (e.g., home healthcare services, medical equipment sales).
   - Provides consulting services for hospitals, clinics, or healthcare organizations.

SETTING PERSONAL AND PROFESSIONAL GROWTH GOALS

To advance in respiratory care leadership, RTs must establish clear goals that align with their career aspirations and personal values.

SMART Goal-Setting Framework

1. Specific – Define clear and precise objectives (e.g., "Become a lead respiratory therapist within two years").
2. Measurable – Establish ways to track progress (e.g., "Complete two leadership training courses this year").
3. Achievable – Set realistic goals based on current skills and opportunities.
4. Relevant – Ensure goals align with career aspirations and personal interests.
5. Time-Bound – Set deadlines to maintain motivation and accountability.

Examples of Personal and Professional Goals

1. Short-Term Goals (1-2 years)
   - Obtain an advanced respiratory therapy certification.
   - Take on a leadership role in a hospital committee.
   - Improve public speaking skills for better team communication.

2. Mid-Term Goals (3-5 years)
   - Transition into a managerial or educator role.
   - Complete a healthcare leadership or business course.
   - Mentor new respiratory therapy graduates.
3. Long-Term Goals (5+ years)
   - Earn a master's degree in healthcare administration.
   - Become a respiratory therapy director or hospital executive.
   - Publish research on innovations in respiratory care.

Leadership development in respiratory care is a lifelong journey that requires dedication, education, mentorship, and goal-setting. Respiratory therapists who actively seek leadership opportunities, engage in professional development, and build strong networks can achieve significant career growth. Whether aspiring to become a department leader, educator, or healthcare administrator, the key to success lies in continuous learning and a commitment to excellence.

By developing leadership skills and advancing their careers, RTs not only enhance their professional lives but also contribute to better patient care and a stronger healthcare system.

DISCUSSION QUESTIONS:

What steps can you take to develop leadership skills in your respiratory care career?

How can mentorship contribute to leadership development in respiratory therapy?

MODULE SIX

CHALLENGES FACED BY LEADERS IN RESPIRATORY CARE AND HOW TO OVERCOME THEM

Leadership in respiratory care comes with unique challenges that require strong problem-solving skills, adaptability, and strategic decision-making. Respiratory therapists (RTs) working in leadership positions must navigate workforce shortages, resistance to change, interdisciplinary conflicts, and financial constraints while ensuring high-quality patient care.

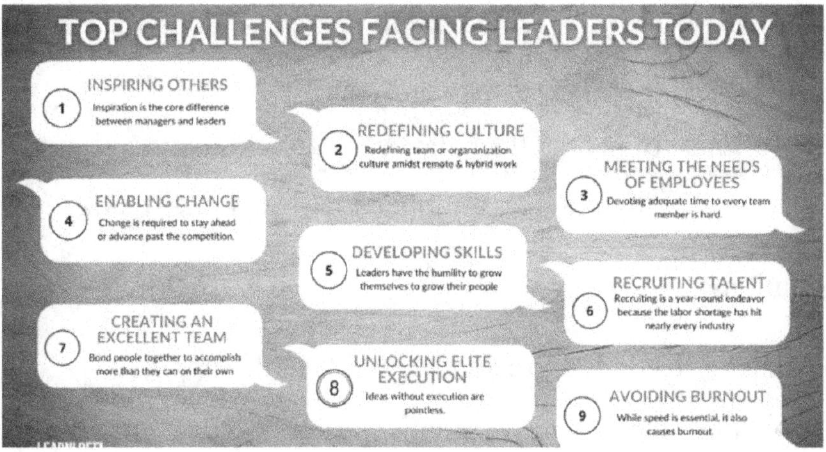
TOP CHALLENGES FACING LEADERS TODAY
1 INSPIRING OTHERS
Inspiration is the core difference between managers and leaders
2 REDEFINING CULTURE
Redefining team or orgaranization culture amidst remote & hybrid work
3 MEETING THE NEEDS OF EMPLOYEES
Devoting adequate time to every team member is hard
4 ENABLING CHANGE
Change is required to stay ahead or advance past the competition
5 DEVELOPING SKILLS
Leaders have the humility to grow themselves to grow their people
6 RECRUITING TALENT
Recruiting is a year-round endeavor because the labor shortage has hit nearly every industry
7 CREATING AN EXCELLENT TEAM
Bond people together to accomplish more than they can on their own
8 UNLOCKING ELITE EXECUTION
Ideas without execution are pointless.
9 AVOIDING BURNOUT
While speed is essential, it also causes burnout

This module explores four significant challenges faced by leaders in respiratory care and provides practical solutions to overcome them.

1. STAFF BURNOUT AND SHORTAGES

The Challenge:

Staff burnout and shortages are among the most pressing issues in healthcare, particularly in respiratory care. RTs often work long hours in high-pressure environments, managing critically ill patients, responding to emergencies, and dealing with emotionally demanding situations. Factors contributing to burnout include:

- High patient loads – A shortage of RTs can lead to excessive workload per staff member.
- Emotional and physical exhaustion – Continuous exposure to critically ill patients and life-or-death situations takes a toll.
- Lack of work-life balance – Rotating shifts, overtime, and being on-call can impact personal well-being.

Solutions:

1. Encourage Self-Care and Mental Health Support
   - Promote wellness initiatives such as stress management workshops, counseling services, and peer support programs.
   - Encourage RTs to take breaks, use vacation time, and maintain a healthy work-life balance.

- Provide access to mindfulness and relaxation techniques, such as meditation or exercise programs.

2. Foster a Supportive Work Environment
   - Recognize and appreciate staff contributions through incentives, awards, or public recognition.
   - Establish open communication channels where employees can voice concerns about workload and stress.
   - Promote teamwork and camaraderie to create a positive workplace culture.
3. Address Staffing Shortages Proactively
   - Advocate for increased hiring and fair staffing ratios to prevent overburdening employees.
   - Offer flexible scheduling options to accommodate work-life balance.
   - Collaborate with educational institutions to encourage students to pursue respiratory therapy careers.
4. Provide Professional Development Opportunities
   - Encourage RTs to take leadership roles, further their education, and participate in specialized training.
   - Create mentorship programs to help newer RTs feel supported and reduce feelings of burnout.

By prioritizing staff well-being and addressing shortages proactively, leaders can reduce burnout and retain a motivated, engaged workforce.

2. RESISTANCE TO CHANGE

The Challenge:

Change is inevitable in healthcare, but not all staff members are receptive to new policies, technologies, or treatment approaches. Resistance to change can arise due to:

- Fear of the unknown – Uncertainty about new techniques or equipment.
- Comfort with existing methods – Long-time employees may prefer traditional practices.
- Lack of understanding – Staff may not see the value in proposed changes.

Solutions:

1. Provide Clear Education and Training
    - Offer hands-on demonstrations, training sessions, and workshops to familiarize staff with new protocols.
    - Explain the benefits of change, such as improved patient outcomes or increased efficiency.
    - Address concerns by providing data, case studies, and expert opinions on the advantages of change.

2. Implement Changes Gradually
    - Avoid overwhelming staff by introducing new policies step by step.
    - Start with pilot programs or small-scale implementations before a full rollout.
    - Encourage staff to provide feedback and make necessary adjustments before finalizing changes.
3. Engage Key Influencers and Early Adopters
    - Identify team members who are open to change and enlist them as champions of new initiatives.
    - When respected colleagues advocate for change, others are more likely to follow.
4. Communicate Effectively and Transparently
    - Leaders should clearly communicate why changes are necessary and how they will benefit both patients and staff.
    - Encourage staff to ask questions and express concerns without fear of judgment.
    - Provide regular updates on the progress of new initiatives.

By fostering a culture of learning and openness, leaders can ease transitions and reduce resistance to change.

3. INTERDISCIPLINARY CONFLICTS

The Challenge:

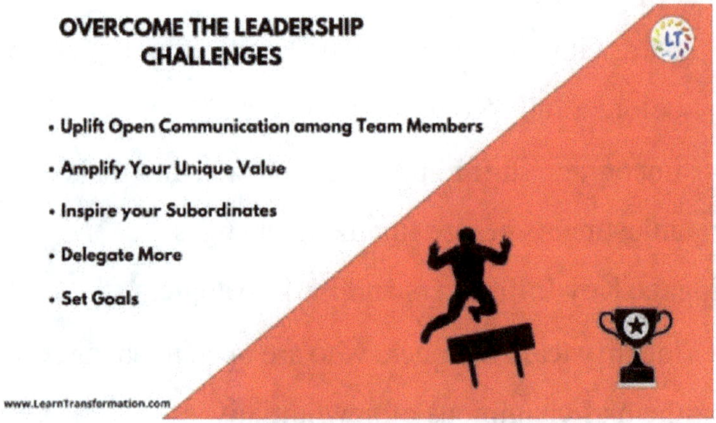
OVERCOME THE LEADERSHIP CHALLENGES
LT
• Uplift Open Communication among Team Members
• Amplify Your Unique Value
• Inspire your Subordinates
• Delegate More
• Set Goals
www.LearnTransformation.com

Respiratory therapists work closely with physicians, nurses, anesthesiologists, and other healthcare professionals. However, differences in roles, communication styles, and decision-making approaches can lead to conflicts, including:

- Miscommunication – Lack of clarity in orders or patient care instructions.
- Role Overlap – Disagreements over responsibilities or scope of practice.
- Varying Priorities – Different healthcare professionals may prioritize tasks differently.

Solutions:

1. Promote Open Dialogue and Teamwork

- Encourage daily interdisciplinary meetings or huddles to discuss patient care plans.
- Foster an environment where all team members feel valued and respected.
- Train RTs in effective communication techniques, such as using structured handoffs (e.g., SBAR – Situation, Background, Assessment, and Recommendation).

2. Establish Clear Roles and Responsibilities
   - Define each team member's role in patient care to avoid confusion or duplication of tasks.
   - Provide ongoing education about the scope of practice for respiratory therapists to ensure understanding among all healthcare providers.
3. Implement Conflict-Resolution Strategies
   - Encourage direct, respectful conversations to address disagreements.
   - Use mediation when necessary to resolve disputes between team members.
   - Promote a problem-solving mindset rather than a blame-focused approach.
4. Encourage Interprofessional Training
   - Organize collaborative training programs that allow different healthcare professionals to learn from one another.

- Encourage cross-disciplinary education to improve understanding and cooperation.

By fostering collaboration and resolving conflicts proactively, leaders can create a more cohesive and efficient healthcare team.

4. BUDGET CONSTRAINTS

The Challenge:

Healthcare facilities often face financial limitations, affecting the availability of resources for respiratory therapy departments. Budget constraints can impact:

- Equipment availability – Limited funding for purchasing or upgrading ventilators, oxygen delivery devices, or diagnostic tools.
- Training and education – Reduced opportunities for staff to attend workshops, conferences, or certification programs.
- Staffing levels – Financial constraints may prevent hiring additional RTs, leading to increased workload.

Solutions:

1. Advocate for Funding and Resource Allocation
    - Present data-driven proposals to hospital administrators outlining the need for additional resources.

- Demonstrate the cost-effectiveness of investing in better equipment and staff training.
- Highlight how adequate funding improves patient outcomes and reduces long-term healthcare costs.

2. Optimize Resource Allocation
    - Prioritize budget spending based on department needs.
    - Implement strategies to reduce waste, such as proper equipment maintenance to extend its lifespan.
    - Consider leasing or refurbishing medical equipment as cost-effective alternatives.
3. Seek External Funding Opportunities
    - Apply for grants and funding programs available for respiratory therapy advancements.
    - Collaborate with medical device companies for sponsorships or research partnerships.
    - Explore government funding or nonprofit support for healthcare initiatives.
4. Implement Cost-Effective Solutions
    - Utilize telehealth or remote monitoring technologies to reduce in-person visits while maintaining patient care quality.
    - Encourage staff cross-training to improve efficiency and reduce the need for additional hiring.

- Leverage online learning platforms for staff education instead of costly in-person training.

By using strategic financial planning and resource management, leaders can overcome budget constraints and continue providing high-quality respiratory care.

Leadership in respiratory care comes with challenges, but proactive problem-solving, strong communication, and strategic decision-making can help overcome them. By addressing burnout and staffing shortages, easing resistance to change, fostering interdisciplinary collaboration, and managing financial constraints effectively, respiratory care leaders can create a sustainable and supportive work environment.

Ultimately, a strong leader is one who continuously learns, adapts, and advocates for both their team and patients. Respiratory therapists who develop leadership skills will not only enhance their careers but also improve the overall quality of respiratory care in healthcare settings.

DISCUSSION QUESTIONS:

What are the most important leadership traits needed for success in respiratory care, and why?

How can respiratory care leaders balance patient advocacy with hospital policies and resource constraints?

CONCLUSION

In this book, we have explored the many dimensions of leadership, from understanding fundamental leadership traits and styles to navigating ethical dilemmas, managing teams, and overcoming challenges unique to respiratory care.

As respiratory therapy continues to evolve with technological advancements, shifting healthcare policies, and increasing patient needs, the demand for strong and adaptable leaders has never been greater. Whether you are a new respiratory therapist looking to develop leadership skills or an experienced professional aiming to refine your approach, effective leadership is within your reach.

The future of respiratory care depends on leaders who are innovative, adaptable, and dedicated to improving patient outcomes. As healthcare systems face new challenges from global pandemics to technological disruptions respiratory therapists must be prepared to step up as leaders, advocates, and change-makers in their field.

By applying the principles discussed in this book, you can strengthen your leadership abilities, inspire your colleagues, and contribute to the advancement of respiratory care. Leadership is not just about directing others; it is about empowering those around you to be their best.

The journey to leadership is ongoing, but every step you take brings you closer to becoming a stronger, more effective, and more compassionate leader.

Now, it is time to take what you have learned and apply it in your daily practice. Lead with confidence, inspire with passion, and always strive for excellence in respiratory care.

REFERENCES

American Association for Respiratory Care (AARC). (2021). *Best practices in respiratory care leadership and management.*

Bass, B. M. (1990). *From transactional to transformational leadership: Learning to share the vision. Organizational Dynamics*, 18(3), 19-31.

Covey, S. R. (1989). *The 7 habits of highly effective people: Powerful lessons in personal change.*

Drucker, P. F. (1999). *Management challenges for the 21st century.* Goleman, D. (1995). *Emotional intelligence: Why it can matter more than IQ*Goleman, D., Boyatzis, R., & McKee, A. (2013). *Primal leadership: Unleashing the power of emotional intelligence.*

Maxwell, J. C. (2005). *The 360-degree leader: Developing your influence from anywhere in the organization.*

McAlearney, A. S. (2010). *Leadership in healthcare: Strategies for effective communication and teamwork.* Northouse, P. G. (2021). *Leadership: Theory and practice (9th ed.).* Spath, P. L. (2018). *Introduction to healthcare quality management (3rd ed.).* Sullivan, E. J. (2017). *Effective leadership and management in nursing (9th ed.)*

Weiss, D., Tilin, F. J., & Morgan, M. J. (2018). The interprofessional health care team: Leadership and development. Jones & Bartlett Learning.

www.ingramcontent.com/pod-product-compliance
Lightning Source LLC
LaVergne TN
LVHW022027200926
848481LV00007B/2568
* 9 7 9 8 3 4 9 2 1 0 1 0 5 *